Katharina Gustavs

Super Breakfast Cereals

Whole grains for good health and great taste

alive books

Vancouver
Canada

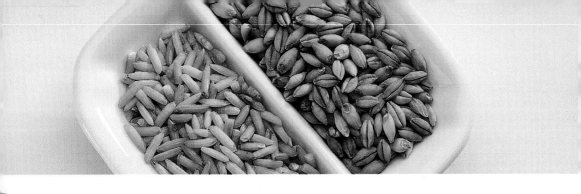

c o n t e n t s

Note: Conversions in this book (from imperial to metric) are not exact. They have been rounded to the nearest measurement for convenience. Exact measurements are given in imperial. The recipes in this book are by no means to be taken as therapeutic. They simply promote the philosophy of both the author and *alive* books in relation to whole foods, health and nutrition, while incorporating the practical advice given by the author in the first section of the book.

Whole Grain Cereal Recipes

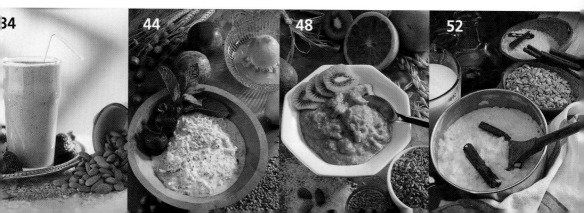

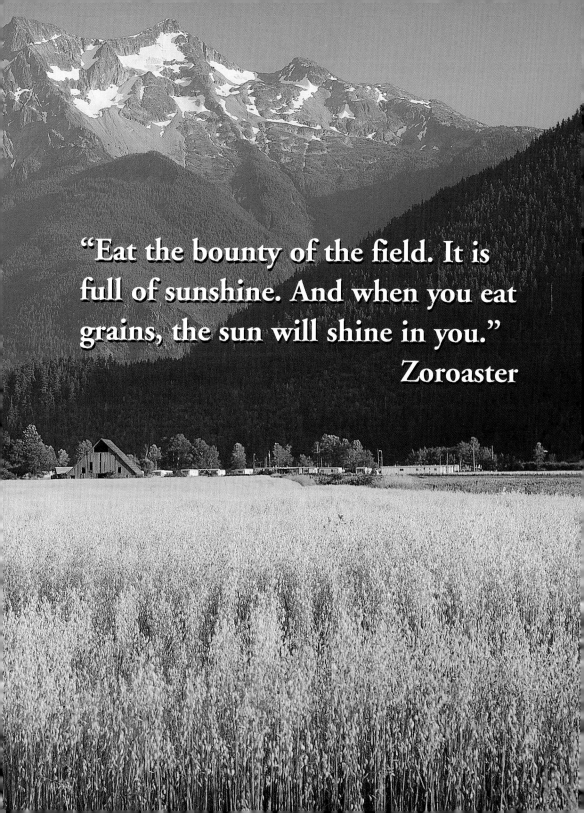

"Eat the bounty of the field. It is full of sunshine. And when you eat grains, the sun will shine in you."

Zoroaster

Introduction . . . .

Whole grains provide energy, promote endurance and are revered worldwide for their life-giving qualities. In fact, whole grains are a worldwide staple food.

For thousands of years humans spared neither trouble nor expense to freshly grind their grains. This smart approach changed only 100 years ago when a whole line of ready-to-eat breakfast cereals sprung up. Since then, savvy advertising, promising health claims and a lack of time have lured many modern homemakers to buy these so-called convenience foods.

At our breakfast table we're offered seemingly wholesome ingredients such as corn, wheat and rice. Yet, processing has changed these ordinary grains to such an extent that your body doesn't recognize or metabolize them any more. Your body cannot efficiently use this so-called food and will send you warning signals—bloating, headaches, allergies, fatigue and more.

In contrast, whole grains provide a natural set of nutrients that your body has been programmed through the ages to metabolize. Eating grains in their whole form will give you essential nutrients such as calcium, magnesium, iron, vitamins E and B complex, enzymes, precious protein, delicate oils, and energy in the form of complex carbohydrates. You can preserve these nutrients by freshly grinding your own grains. As soon as you crack

Whole grains provide a natural set of nutrients that your body can efficiently use.

M. Kellar, First Light

6

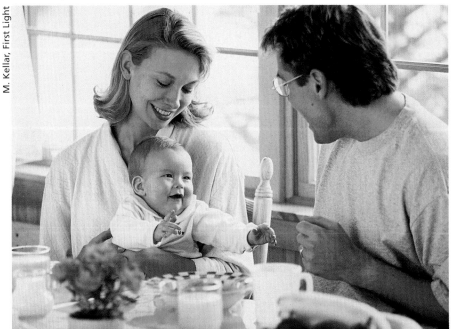

open whole grains their delicate nutrients will start to deteriorate and rancidity occurs. Eating them frequently milled, instead of processed and rancid, will provide both taste and health benefits.

When I was a child, I loved to stay with my grandmother who lived in the mountains surrounded by wild creeks, spruce forests and large oat fields. She taught me the healing powers of many plants while foraging for mushrooms and berries. During August we would eat oats, freshly plucked from the field. What a sweet taste! After a long day's work and just before going to bed, grandmother would fill her hand mill with her favorite grains and grind them for a fresh raw breakfast dish. Once you've smelled freshly ground grains, you won't settle for anything else.

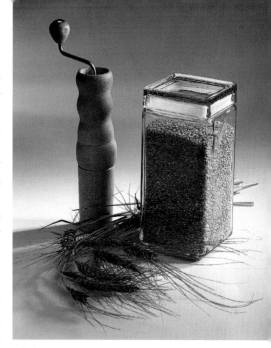

The hand mill makes a favorite, fresh, raw breakfast possible.

Nobody will dispute the delicious and satisfying feeling you get from eating a freshly picked and fully ripe apple. At its best, natural sweetness is so sublime that we make great efforts to grow fruit ourselves or obtain local fruit from a nearby farmer. Why settle for less when buying cereal grains? They were called "fruit of the field" in the ancient past.

When left whole in nature's original packaging, cereal grains offer a great advantage over any fruit or vegetable. Because they travel far without spoilage and store well until the next harvest, you can always have them on hand: fresh, sweet and nourishing– as long as you leave them whole. Grind, crack or flake them only when you're ready for them and all their goodness will open up to you. All you need to get started is a grain mill.

Today, many people think milled whole grains are tasteless and boring. But that's because these grains, from the supermarket and even health stores, are already rancid by the time you prepare and eat them. The good news is that you don't have to buy your grains in this fashion. You can buy whole grains and mill them easily yourself. Today, it's easier than ever to enjoy freshly ground grains for breakfast.

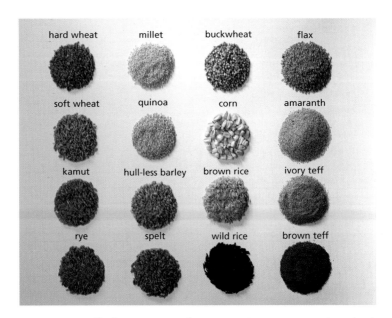

hard wheat   millet   buckwheat   flax

soft wheat   quinoa   corn   amaranth

kamut   hull-less barley   brown rice   ivory teff

rye   spelt   wild rice   brown teff

Grain mills have come a long way since my grandmother's days and now modern machines will help you prepare grains in a flash. So why shortchange yourself at breakfast, the most important meal of the day? Once you're in the habit of grinding your own grains, you'll experience better health and have loads of energy to spare. Rancid, processed cereals that smells like paint thinner and taste like sawdust will be a thing of the past.

How Healthy Are Common Breakfast Cereals?

The convenience of ready-to-eat breakfast cereals is tempting. Preparation time is reduced to zero, but what if the nutritional value also converges toward zero? Did you ever wonder why a whole wheat cereal is fortified with iron even though wheat bran, normally bursting with natural iron, is in the ingredients? Cereal manufacturers add wheat bran to provide roughage, which is good for us, but having over-processed leftover bran dumped into our bowls is not necessarily a healthy choice. And a "fat free" claim only indicates that the manufacturer withholds precious germ oils.

In the 1970s, American researchers fed rats common breakfast cereals, all of which were enriched with the most important vitamins and minerals. Instead of rearing rats vibrating with good health, these tough laboratory breeds came down with anemia, fatty livers and high blood pressure. They were close to death. If cereal designed to meet current scientific nutritional requirements can bring rats close to death, it can't be doing much for your health? Obviously, denatured processed food cannot be revived with an overload of synthetic vitamins and minerals–nor can it sustain us. We still have a lot to learn about the complex nature of our metabolism.

The proof seems to be in the pot. Cooking grains in an ordinary pot takes time, and so the cereal food industry invented a magic pot, the so-called extruder, which uses unnaturally high pressure and heat to minimize processing time and, by the way, maximize profits. The results are nicely shaped bits that look tempting to the eye, but are foreign to the body. Today unfortunately, most cereal flake, organic or non-organic, is cooked this way.

Why Whole Grains? . . . .

There is wisdom in the way plants grow. The whole grain package of germ, bran and endosperm is designed to go together, and the various components aid each other in the digestion of the whole. Processing and refining takes apart this package, resulting in significant nutrient loss. And when you leave something out, you risk developing imbalances due to missing nutrients and incomplete metabolism.

The whole is more than the sum of its parts.

Processing the Nutrients Out of Wheat			
	Whole Wheat Kernel (per 100 g)	White Wheat Flour (per 100 g)	% Lost
Calcium	44 mg	15 mg	66%
Iron	3.3 mg	1.9 mg	42%
Magnesium	147 mg	20 mg	86%
Potassium	502 mg	108 mg	78%
Vitamin E	1400 mg	400 mg	71%
Vitamin B$_1$	480 mg	60 mg	87%
Folic acid	49 mg	10 mg	80%

(Source: Karl von Koerber, Thomas Männle and Claus Leitzmann. Heidelberg: Vollwert-Ernährung, 1994.)

In our analytical times, we're obsessed with separating almost everything into its component parts in order to understand its true nature. Whole cereal grains are no exception. The most vital ingredients were taken from whole grains before reaching an understanding of their synergetic relationship and benefits. Recent scientific studies have come to the same conclusion as our ancestors: *Whole cereal grains are nature's most complete food package.*

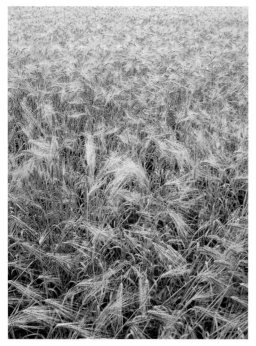

The ancient grain barley is particularly rich in silica and has strengthening, soothing, and cholesterol-lowering properties.

Don't be fooled. The whole is more than the sum of its components. Start with whole grains in their wholesome form as grown in the field. Don't trust food manufacturers who first process all the goodness out of the grain in order to put back their synthetic concoctions according to "scientifically" proven formulas. Sun-grown bounty is still the best food for you.

Start simply; don't start with a multi-grain cereal. Give your body a chance to explore each grain on its own before you combine different ones. Each grain in itself is packed with a multidimensional spectrum of nutrients. There are so many marvelous grains, and you need not have them all in one single spoonful. Taste for yourself and enjoy good health.

Raw Cereals–A Fresh Impulse . . . .

While most sprouted grains need gentle heat to render them more easily digestible, a few are suitable for eating raw on a regular basis. Oat groats (hulled or crushed oats) are the notable exception. Wheat sprouts and buckwheat are also great options. Some naturopaths suggest eating a raw soaked 7-grain cereal to boost the immune system. (Medicine doesn't have to taste bitter, and especially for grains, bitterness indicates rancidity, which challenges our liver to detoxify.)

The first grass seeds ever eaten were certainly fresh from the field. In order to meet your nutritional needs, however, you would have to spend close to a whole day chewing a handful of these grains. Even sprouted grains take a long time to chew thoroughly. Thank goodness it didn't take long for humans to invent the quern (a hand mill), which was soon followed by the quick-and-easy raw breakfast cereal. Soft, nutritious and delicious, mush was not just for babies back then–and it doesn't have to be today. In the Carpathian Mountains in Poland, for example, the Goralen people still enjoy eating their oatmeal raw.

The advantages of raw food are obvious and manifold, as all heat-sensitive nutrients remain intact. The abundance of live enzymes restores tired bodies and stressed minds. However, raw cereal grains can overtax our bodies. Even though soaking and sprouting converts a lot of the grain's complex carbohydrates resulting in easy digestion, a certain amount always remains that proves a bit too complex for our system. Therefore, if you experience trouble digesting raw whole grains (soaked meal or sprouted kernels), you should consume them in small amounts or reserve them for therapeutic use. You can get your nutrients and enzymes by eating other, more suitable raw foods throughout the day.

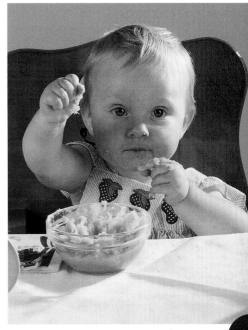

Oats help prevent infections and contagious diseases in children because they are a natural internal antiseptic.

To benefit optimally from raw cereals, always crack your whole grains and seeds-freshly. Only then will natural sweetness and new vitality reward you. With just a little preparation, raw breakfast cereals are incredibly easy to make–see the recipe section for simple and delicious raw-grain cereals.

Hot Cereals–A Comfort Food . . . .

It didn't take our ancestors long to figure out that gentle heat works wonders on whole grains. People who left the tropics and tried to withstand cold winters learned to appreciate the comforting quality of hot whole grain cereal.

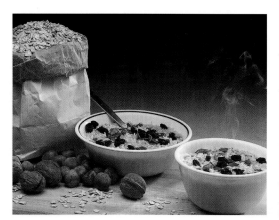

The humble porridge gives you endurance through its heart-warming and soul-satisfying qualities.

A handful of grains, soaked then gently simmered and heated, delivers warmth and strength in a most soothing way. Tribes throughout the world developed their own preference for certain grains–depending on availability, and for specific grinds–depending on individual taste buds. Scots, for example, love their oatmeal ground fine to coarse, while the Irish prefer them steel-cut. The English and Americans use mainly rolled oats. People in Southern Germany revere spelt, an ancient variety of wheat, never quite understanding why others bother with ordinary wheat. Greek philosophers swore by their barley and Asians never tire of eating rice three times a day.

Despite the popularity of fast-food restaurants, plain hot cereal is still the most-eaten food around the world. The most basic version is called gruel, which usually evokes images of the poor, surviving on a watery soup that barely nourishes. Poor or rich aside, the first image of gruel is accurate–ground meal is simmered in a lot of water. However, the truth of whether it's barely nourishing depends on what type of ground meal is used.

White flour, of course, doesn't nourish at all. It is stripped of much of its composition so it will deteriorate machine processing. The end result is a flour that contains almost no nutritional value. Wholemeal is a step in the right direction, but it must be freshly ground otherwise its nutrients are lost through oxidation. And for all the "poor" people whose digestive systems are overworked by processed food, gruel is a good introduction to whole grain food.

Freshly grinding grains makes the bran more easily digestible, pre-soaking makes all the minerals available and gentle simmering breaks up the complex starch. Incorporating these steps into your daily routine is easy to do and it will lead to better health. Try one cereal grain at a time and see how you react to it. The humble porridge, be it thick or thin, will give you endurance through its heart-warming and soul-satisfying qualities.

Cold Cereals–Adding Some Crunch . . . .

It's only natural for people leading busy and fast-paced lives to seek out convenience foods like ready-to-eat breakfast cereals. Don't rely on the food industry, however, to deliver nutritious foods. Whatever they cook up in their magic pot is better left untouched.

It's worthwhile to create your own crunchy treats by popping grains in a frying pan. Commercial puffed cereal consists of grains shot from guns under extreme pressure. Laboratory rats died after a two-week diet of commercial puffed wheat.

We're not the first ones to look for food that travels well and is quick to prepare. In South America, cattle-herders discovered that slowly dry-toasted grains were the perfect food for sustaining them over long trips. The time needed to prepare their meals was reduced immensely. Plus, dry-toasted whole grains, prepared accordingly, are quite easy to digest.

Those who don't like mushy cereal can add some crunch by flaking, cracking or popping their cereal grains. Traditional dry-toasting allows you to store cereal for roughly four months and have them conveniently ready to go.

Muesli means "soft food," but today stands for a crunchy mixture of rolled oats, nuts, and dried fruit. Store-bought varieties

Unsulphured, dried fruit is a wonderful, healthful addition to cereal.

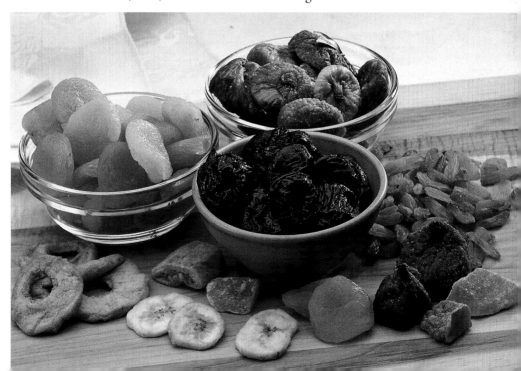

are known for their staleness and rancidity. In the form of granola, this otherwise harmless mixture becomes downright toxic through the application of very high temperatures and the addition of hydrogenated fats, not to mention all the sugar. It's best to mix your own muesli.

> When making your own muesli, purchase unsulphured fruit. Fresh nuts, although a bit more difficult to find, are also wonderful for both taste and health, and are well worth the search.

In the recipe section you'll find many ideas to create your own raw, hot or cold breakfast cereals full of nutrients and packed with live energy. It doesn't take a lot of extra time to start your cereals from scratch, just a bit of planning. Prepared with love and eaten with joy, breakfast can be a celebration of life. Keep it simple and goodness will follow you throughout the day.

Buying Whole Grains . . . .

Local health food stores usually carry a large selection of whole grains and you can often order a 55-pound or 25-pound bag and receive a 10 to 15 percent discount. You can also order directly from farmers or reliable milling operations. As a general rule, grains in paper bags are usually fresher because they're not subject to light during storage.

When buying, follow these guidelines and you'll benefit from the most life-giving grains possible.

Buy Organic

It wasn't that long ago when all food was simply grown organically. These days, organic foods, including certified organically grown grains, are a specialty crop.

Organic seeds are not genetically altered so that your body can recognize and metabolize them properly. The grains are grown, handled and stored without the use of synthetic chemicals, which are known to wreak havoc with our system–if not right away then definitely in the long term. The mineral content in organic crops is higher compared to "regular" crops, so your body will be filled and actually nourished. And the superior electrochemical quality of truly organic crops provides the life-energy required for vibrant health.

High Germination Rate

Whole grains are basically seeds. As long as they maintain the capacity to sprout, grains are more resistant to any type of spoilage and offer the highest nutritional value since they still contain all vital nutrients. Less than 80 percent sprouted kernels is not worth eating and such a batch of grains is not considered a whole food by leading experts.

Check the "Sproutability" of Your Grains

It's important to check the sproutability of the grains you buy. Simply soak 100 kernels of wheat, for instance, in one cup (250 ml) of water overnight. Drain them the next morning and rinse them twice daily for the next two to three days. Then count the number of kernels that actually grow a little shoot.

100 sprouted kernels is ideal
90 sprouted kernels is good
85 sprouted kernels is fair

Optimal Dryness

Whole grains must be dry for storage and for grinding. The moisture content of the grain is a crucial factor–if the grain is too moist, it will turn moldy during storage and jam your grain mill during grinding. An ideal moisture content is 12 to 14 percent. Your grains should feel dry to the touch. If in doubt, put your nose in a handful of grains to tell whether they smell moist and moldy.

Cleanness

Only properly cleaned whole grains are fit for human consumption. Don't tolerate any mold or pests in your grains, and any foreign materials, damaged kernels and dust should be rare. You should even check the quality of your so-called germ-free and vacuum-sealed grains.

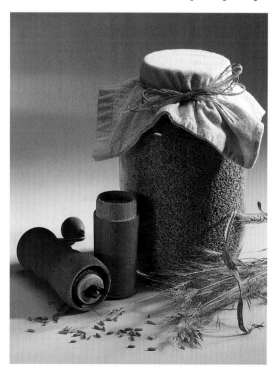

Whole grains must be dry for both storage and grinding.

15

A Cereal Grain for Everyone

A large selection of grains is available year round. Familiarize yourself with a variety of grains and seeds and choose the ones that best fit your constitution and state of health. Besides the seven families of true grains (barley, corn, millet, oat, rice, rye, and wheat), other botanical families (amaranth, buckwheat, and goosefoot) produce seeds that can be eaten just like grains.

Amaranth Family: A tiny seed bursting with abundant goodness, amaranth, Greek for "not withering," lives up to its name–resisting heat and drought to sprout even after decades of dormancy. The Aztecs revered this crop for its magical powers and mixed it with blood on holy days. Amaranth contains a balance of proteins and more calcium than cow's milk.

Barley Family: Possibly the earliest cereal grain, barley was cultivated as far back as 9,000 ago. Greek philosophers considered barley the ultimate brain food because it increased alertness, and Roman gladiators were called "barley eaters" because eating this marvelous grain gave them strength. In modern times, barley is prized for its outstanding cholesterol-lowering properties as well as for its popular role in making beer. Pearl barley is stripped of vital nutrients. A hull-less variety is your best bet.

Buckwheat Family: Buckwheat incorporated "wheat" in its name and can be cooked like wheat, but the resemblance ends there. Originally grown in Mongolia and Nepal, buckwheat became a staple in Russia and Eastern Europe. It contains more of the amino acid lysine than most grains, and it combines well with other grains. Roasted buckwheat groats are called kasha, after the famous Russian gruel, and if you love the peculiar taste of these roasted groats, make sure they are dry-toasted without any fat.

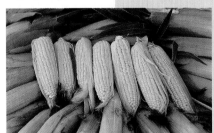

Corn provides a wide range of vitamins and minerals, and contains high quality protein.

Corn Family: Corn is a true native of the Americas, endowing the indigenous people with enormous strength and endurance. Unfortunately, most versions of the ready-to-eat cereal made out of corn (cornflake) are pushed through an extruder, resulting in a final product that's devoid of bioavailable nutrients, no matter how it is "enriched." Only traditional yellow corn or heirloom varieties such as blue corn provide rich nourishment.

Goosefoot Family (Quinoa): The Incas called quinoa (pronounced "keen-wa") "the mother grain" and it is packed with protein, calcium, and much more to boost energy. The best variety is still grown high up in the Andes and these seeds of pale ivory taste sweet and succulent. Bitter-tasting, dark-colored seeds are of the poorest grade grown at sea level. Since quinoa is coated with saponin to preserve freshness, you must thoroughly rinse the bitterness out of it.

Millet Family: The millet family comes in many forms and sizes, including such exotics as Job's tears from Asia and teff from Ethiopia. We usually see a golden-colored millet. Its high silicon content nourishes and beautifies skin, hair and nails, and it is a popular choice for overactive children and stressed adults due to its alkali-forming nature and easy digestibility. Most millet, however, tastes bitter because its germ oils have deteriorated with the dehulling process. To restore its delicate taste and nutritional value, wash millet with hot water and rinse several times with cold water.

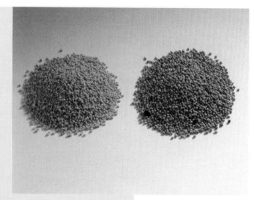

Millet, shown here hull-less and hulled, was an important staple food in Biblical times, and is considered sacred in China.

Oat Family: Oat was a staple food of the Celtic and Germanic people, who were known for their physical strength. Oat is considered an excellent remedy for upset stomach and over-stressed nerves, providing an abundance of minerals, vitamins, mucilage and fat, as well as a hormone-like stimulant. Hot steam is commonly used to loosen oat groat hulls prior to hulling and unfortunately this heat treatment causes the oats to lose their ability to sprout. To enjoy the sweetness of raw oats, find a supplier who can offer oats that are not heat-treated or you may want to hull them yourself using a grain flaker. I also recommend seeking out the "naked" variety in the oat family (referred to as a hull-less variety) as its threshing usually doesn't involve heat. Always eat a few oat groats before buying. They should taste pleasant and sweet, not bitter.

Rice Family: Instead of saying, "How are you?" Asians ask, "Did you have your rice today?" Though the nutrients in rice aren't found in especially high amounts, their quality is indisputable. Its composition of sodium and potassium, for example, benefits the kidney with a dewatering effect. Rice comes in long, medium and short sizes and almost any color. Buy the whole kernel, as in brown rice, and avoid parboiled or polished versions.

Rye Family: The first Europeans brought along wheat as well as rye to North America. While the wheat withered away in the harsh new climate, the hardy rye took root. The roots of rye plants reach amazingly deep into the earth and deliver a vast array of minerals for our benefit. Its high potassium content, for instance, is soothing for the liver. Rye is perfectly matched with authentic sourdough, and its creamy consistency lends itself to a comforting hot cereal.

Wheat Family: Wheat is grown all over the world. It isn't by chance that we crave wheat since its nutritional profile is quite similar to that of the human body. Wheat balances and calms the heart and mind. More and more people seem to be wheat-intolerant, which in many cases is caused by genetically altered strains or rancidity. Spelt, soft wheat and kamut are good choices for breakfast cereal.

Check your grains to avoid the following:

mold • pests • rancidity • staleness • grain dust • foreign materials

Color Check

Darker spots and speckles	Might indicate mold. The color of grains naturally varies a lot even within a given batch.
Dark purple, almost black kernels of double size	Indicate ergot, a piece of toxic fungus usually found in rye or wheat varieties. Even though it takes about 150 kernels of ergot at one meal to induce toxic effects, any pieces should be removed.
White patches	Indicate utilized starch, which means that the nutrients have been used up already.

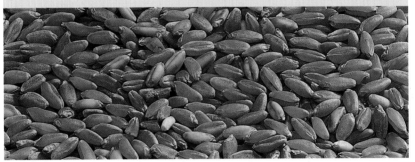

Pest Check

Round holes in individual kernels	Indicate grain weevils.
Mass of eggs and excrement webbed together	Indicate flour moth.
Huge amounts of grain dust	Indicate grain mite.

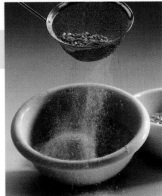

18

Odor Check

Moldy or fishy smell

Indicates mold. Certain mycotoxins produced by mold are among the most powerful toxins known to humans. However, you will not always discover visible signs of mold.

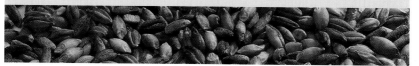

Acidic smell

Indicates bacteria.

Rancid smell (like foul eggs or paint thinner)

Indicates rancidity. The husking or hulling process exposed the delicate germ oils to oxygen, resulting in peroxides, which are hard on the liver.

Stale smell

Indicates improper storage and/or old age.

Foreign Material Check

Foreign seeds

Are mainly weed seeds. They tend to take longer to cook and taste bitter, but are usually harmless.

Tiny rocks and dirt lumps

Need to be removed to save your teeth and milling heads from trouble.

Bits of husks

Should be rare.

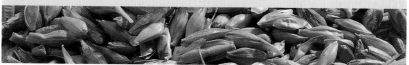

Damaged grains

Should be rare. They tend to be rancid.

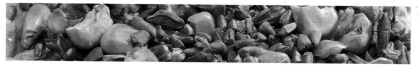

Storing Whole Grains . . . .

Whole grains are living food and a whole lot of other living creatures—not just humans—want to eat them. Therefore proper storage is inevitable to keep away other hungry creatures and to prevent spoilage. In short, grains need to be stored in a dry, cool, and dark place. Under optimal conditions, you can easily store whole grains for years with little nutrient loss.

Dry, Cool, and Dark

Successfully storing whole grains depends in particular on their moisture content. The drier the grains (below 12 percent moisture content), the better they will keep. Even though grains are in a dormant state, they need to breathe and appreciate resting in a well-ventilated place. Excellent storage choices are wooden boxes, paper or linen bags, or glass jars with breathable lids. If you feel safer about using glass jars with an airtight lid, always leave an air space of about 1 to 2 inches (2 to 5 cm) on top and make sure you open the jars at least once a month.

Larger amounts (55-pound or 25-kg bags and higher), however, should not be stored in rooms where the humidity level fluctuates a great deal (such as your kitchen) because the grains might absorb too much moisture over a lengthy period. Simply put them in a grain chest made of solid wood, which is a great buffer for fluctuating humidity levels.

Store dry grains in a well-ventilated place in wooden boxes, paper or linen bags, or glass jars with breathable lids.

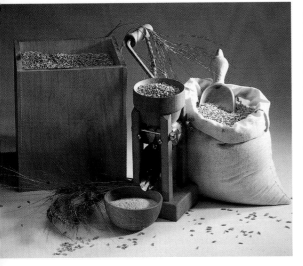

A temperature of 53°F (12°C) is ideal for storing whole grains. It is not necessary to put grains in the refrigerator. Fortunately, when the grains are dry (below 12 percent moisture content), the temperature for storing them can range tremendously and they will even keep well at room temperature over a long period. The occasional summer heat won't hurt.

In their dry state, grains are kind of hibernating: still alive, but metabolizing at a very, very low rate. Since light usually speeds up life processes, grains exposed to light lose vital

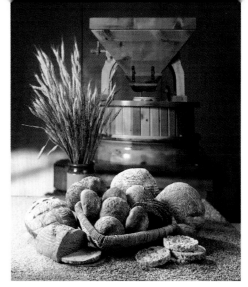

nutrients faster. Therefore it is important to store grains in dark containers such as wooden boxes or paper or linen bags. If you put them in clear glass jars, you should store these in a cupboard and not in the open.

If you don't plan on using large amounts of grain within a month, it is imperative to stir the grain every six to eight weeks in order to disrupt the grain weevil's growth cycle and prevent any spoilage.

Choosing Grain Mills and Flakers · · · · · · · · · ·

The only thing standing between you and freshly milled grains is a grain mill or flaker. There are a wide range of options for purchasing and all and any effort made to eat freshly milled whole grains will be priceless when it comes to taste and health.

Investing in a grain mill or flaker will provide the priceless results of taste and health.

The perfect mill doesn't require a lot of space yet holds a lot of flour. It consumes no electricity yet grinds huge amounts of grains. It doesn't create noise, dust or heat, and will never wear out. It looks beautiful and costs very little. This mill has yet to be invented.

Meanwhile, it is important to choose a mill that best suits your family's needs. A large selection of grain mills is available, and no matter which one you acquire, your freshly ground flour or cracked meal will always taste much better than any pre-packaged store-bought grain. It's even worthwhile to use a blender to freshly grind the softer varieties such as oats, millet, buckwheat, and amaranth.

Hand Mills

In ancient times the first grains were crushed in a mortar or rubbed in a quern. Today, any hand-operated mill is still a treasure because it will mill despite a power outage and travel wherever you go. Hand mills are the best and most gentle choice for grinding grain, because the slower the grinding, the better it is for the grain. The disadvantage of hand mills, however, is that they require a great deal of manpower.

A hand mill is a good place to start exploring whole grain food before you invest in an electric grain mill. In most cases, though, the slow-grinding crank will probably speed up your decision to purchase an electric mill. Some hand mills offer the option of hooking it up to a motor.

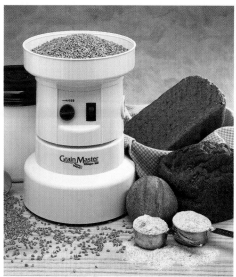

With an electric mill you can grind whole grains quickly, easily, and whenever you need them.

Electric Mills

Electric mills offer the great advantage of freshly grinding your grains whenever, and however much, you need–no matter how big your family.

The milling heads of the various models are mostly made out of steel or stone. Steel burrs are versatile because you can also grind a whole range of oily seeds such as nuts and beans, even though they tend to produce a rather coarse flour. Stone milling heads produce very fine and fluffy flour and, unlike the steel burrs, do not heat up during milling.

There are also mills that do not grind, but rather burst the grain using microburst technology, a process developed by the pharmaceutical industry to create uniform particles for use in medicine. Grinding is always stressful to the grain and microbursting seems to create the most stress. Remember, the slower the grinding, the better.

A kitchen machine with a grain mill attachment is an economical choice. However, keep in mind that an attachment requires precious time to set up the various components. For daily use, you will appreciate a permanent solution, a machine that you can just turn on and grind. Consider these features when looking for an electric grain mill:

- The setting from coarse to fine is clearly marked and easily adjustable.
- The ground flour is collected without developing a lot of dust.
- The mill can be switched on and off during milling operation.
- The mill and milling heads clean easily, even if it has a self-cleaning chamber.

- Industrial motors perform best because they are designed to withstand continuous strain, gumming, and jamming.
- Look for motors with a low sound level; industrial motors seem to make the least noise.
- Make sure the mill doesn't heat the flour too much; flour temperature should be below 104°F (40°C). As a general rule, the slower the grain mill, the better. The faster the grain mill, the faster it will destroy heat-sensitive vitamins and enzymes. A mill with a cooling system, however, provides the benefit of a very low-temperature flour.
- The least aeration created by the milling operation is desirable, in order to keep oxidation rate low.
- Check with the supplier to ensure the mill grinds tiny grains such as amaranth or hard grains such as corn.

Grain Flakers

You can roll your own oats, and other cereal grains, with a grain flaker (which is also know as a roller). Usually a hand flaker will suffice, however, there are attachments for grain mills available as well. I prefer steel rollers because they can handle moist grains and oily seeds and are easy to clean. Stone rollers are also an option. Grain flakers are great for cracking grains if you prefer a chewier texture. The hopper easily holds 1 cup (250 ml) of grains. Be sure cereal flakes don't spill out during the flaking process.

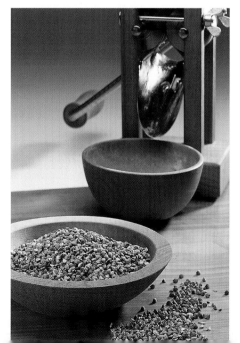

A grain flaker or roller is excellent for rolling oats and other cereal grains.

Preparing Whole Grains . . . .

It is important to start with the best quality whole grains. Then it's your preparation method that determines whether you'll have a healthy feast or an unhealthy, bad-tasting experience. The following traditional preparation methods have been developed through the simple holistic lifestyle of days gone by and gut-tested over thousands of years rather than analyzed in laboratories. Recent scientific findings continue to confirm the wisdom of these traditions. For instance, the more you pre- and post-soak, the less your grain dish will be acid-forming, and the healthier it is for you.

Pre-Soaking

Any preparation of whole grains ideally starts with soaking them in cold water, regardless of whether you're using whole kernels or wholemeal. Soak time depends on the size or grind–somewhere between 15 minutes (fine flour) and 10 hours (whole kernels). The temperature should be kept between 50°F (10°C) to 68°F (20°C)–not too cold or too hot–to allow beneficial enzymatic reactions to occur.

The water combined with the right temperature triggers a whole host of biochemical reactions, making all the nutrients available to begin the plant's new life. This type of bioavailability is also imperative for human digestion.

Some people put soaked grains in the refrigerator, for fear that soaking promotes too many germs. However, enzymes as well as germs are too cold in the refrigerator and any desired enzymatic reactions will be "frozen." As usual, the truth is in the balance. Some germs are always present and usually won't harm (unless you've developed a microbial imbalance), but rather exercise and strengthen your immunity. The enzymes react at temperatures that are generally safe for background germs to naturally occur, provided that the soak time is limited to ten hours and no pathogenic microbes are present in the first place.

Soak grains or wholemeal only in water and always on their own. Soak any dried fruit separately. When soaking whole kernels, cover them with water; when soaking wholemeal, make sure it resembles a thick pancake batter with no water collecting on its surface.

Pre-Soaking Times for Whole Grains	
Grains	**Pre-soak Time**
Fine flour or small grains e.g., millet, buckwheat, amaranth, quinoa	15 minutes
Coarse meal, flakes or medium grains e.g., brown rice, oats	1-3 hours
Whole kernels e.g., wheat, rye, barley	3-10 hours

Sprouting

Sprouts contain more live enzymes and energy than any other food. You can easily grow grains at home to yield small sprouts for a delicious vital cereal.

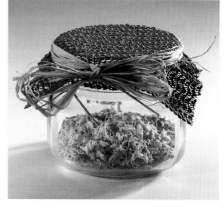

After pre-soaking a batch of viable whole kernels, simply pour off the soak water and let the seeds sprout, in the dark and at room temperature, in a clay saucer or a jar covered with a screen (cheese cloth or a jay cloth is fine). Rinse the sprouts with fresh water two to three times daily. Once they are ready to eat, most grain sprouts are best lightly steamed. Bitter-tasting sprouts were grown beyond their prime.

Whole grains may also be sprouted for an especially healthful and energizing cereal or salad.

Dry-Toasting

Dry-toasted grains can be ground into flour, which will keep for about four months with negligible nutrient loss when stored properly. However, if you first grind the grain and then dry-toast it, just for the nutty flavor, it won't keep very well, and is not easily digested. The minimal pre-soaking makes all the difference for optimal digestibility and keeping quality, and it makes the flour sweeter–naturally.

First, rinse the cereal grains until the water runs clear. Place rinsed grains in a ceramic or glass bowl and cover with a lid. Over the next one to ten hours, the moisture from rinsing will be absorbed through the outer layers of bran, initiating the biochemical reactions described in the pre-soaking process.

Dry-toasted whole grains will keep for approximately four months.

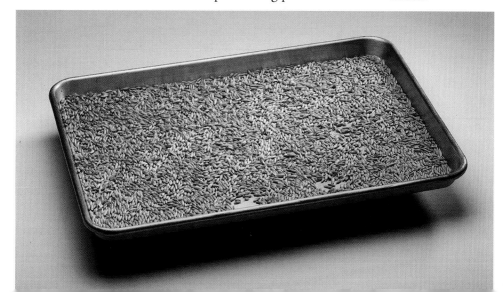

Once the grains feel almost dry to the touch, spread them evenly on a large baking sheet and place them in the oven. Set the temperature from 175°F (80°C) to 250°F (100°C). It takes about one to two hours to dry grains thoroughly, depending on their moisture content. An aromatic scent and a golden hue will indicate that toasting is finished. Roasting is not desired.

Place dry-toasted grains in an airtight container and store at room temperature for up to 4 months. These grains are handy for making quick-and-easy muesli or granola.

Flaking

Both of the following methods will produce freshly rolled flakes that are best consumed the same day or can be refrigerated for a few days in airtight containers. If you want to use them even later, preserve them by dry-toasting, preferably after flaking with the moist method.

Dry Method: First, put dry grains through a flaker. Hard grains such as wheat, barley, and rye will only crack, more so in a

hand flaker than an electric one. Oat groats when rolled will resemble a flake, due to their high fat content. Smaller grains and seeds will be just crushed. Your next step is to pre-soak (see "Pre-Soaking," page 28).

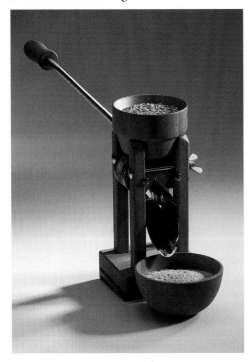

Moist Method: First, rinse the cereal grains until the water runs clear. Place rinsed grains in a ceramic or glass bowl and cover with a lid. Over the next one to ten hours, the moisture from rinsing will be absorbed through the outer layers of bran, initiating the biochemical reactions described in the pre-soaking process. Once the grains feel almost dry to the touch, put them through a flaker and turn out nicely shaped flakes.

Simmering

Grain simmered in water gelatinizes the starch. Water molecules break up long chains of complex carbohydrates, rendering them available for human digestion. Cell walls are also broken down and made more easily digestible.

Since enzymes cannot withstand the heat from simmering, it is important to pre-soak whole grains so that respective enzymes can do their job–for example releasing valuable minerals–before they're destroyed by the heat. Any time you pour whole grains or their meal into a pot of boiling water, the abundance of minerals from the bran layers will, at best, pass unabsorbed and be lost. In the worst case, the phytochemicals in the grain's lock-in mechanism will throw off your whole mineral balance.

Heat sufficient water in a pot and add *pre-soaked* kernels, flakes or wholemeal. Bring the mixture to a simmer then turn down the heat to low and gently simmer for five to ten minutes for fine flour or small grains, approximately twenty minutes for coarse meal or medium grains, or one to three hours for hardy whole kernels.

Simmering Times for Whole Grains	
Grain	**Simmer Time**
Fine flour or small grains e.g., millet, buckwheat, amaranth, quinoa	5-10 minutes
Coarse meal, flakes or medium grains e.g., brown rice, oats	20 minutes
Whole kernels e. g., wheat, rye, barley	1-3 hours

Double boilers, rice cookers and crock pots are ideal for cooking grains because the buffer zone of hot water or air around the grains prevents sticking. There are stainless steel, high-tech rice cookers on the market, which can be programmed to cook 1 to 10 cups of grain at a specific time and temperature. An ordinary rice cooker will also work, as long as it is made out of stainless steel or ceramic and not out of plastic or aluminum. Crock pots with ceramic bowls are available, and some of them also have an additional "keep warm" setting. Stainless steel double boilers or simmer pots are versatile and easy to use and are also available in glass.

Post-Soaking

Post-soaking your cereal completes the gelatinization process. Keep the pot just hot–not boiling–between 140°F (60°C) and 175°F (80°C) to allow for a slow and gentle process. Post-soak times range from twenty minutes to three hours. Here a double boiler or a rice cooker comes in handy.

When you turn off the heat, place an unbleached cotton or paper towel under the lid to catch the condensation. In the past people used to have dough boxes or simply wrapped a woolen blanket around their pot of porridge to keep it warm.

Post-Soaking Times for Whole Grains	
Grain	**Post-soak Time**
Fine flour or small grains e.g., millet, buckwheat, amaranth, quinoa	20-30 minutes
Coarse meal, flakes, or medium grains e.g., brown rice, oats	30-60 minutes
Whole kernels e.g., wheat, rye, barley	1-3 hours

Cooking While You Sleep: Timing Your Hot Cereal

Don't forgo the energy and comfort of your morning hot cereal because you're in a rush. Enjoying a quick-and-easy breakfast is simply a matter of letting the grains come to life while you sleep.

Stove-Top Method: Grind the cereal grain of your choice in the evening, let it soak overnight, and cook it first thing in the morning. If you're in a hurry, grind the grain the previous afternoon for pre-soaking, cook it in the evening, and let it post-soak all night in a warm place. If desired, gently reheat the porridge the next morning, adding more hot water until the desired consistency.

Crock Pot Method: If you don't own a grain mill, simply pre-soak the whole kernels of your choice a little longer during the day, from one to four hours up to ten hours. That evening, simmer grain in lots of water in a slow cooker, rice cooker or crock pot for one to two hours. When you go to bed, turn down to "keep warm." In the morning this breakfast cereal will welcome you with comforting warmth. If desired, run it through a blender for a smoother texture.

Thermos Bottle Method: Place one of the fast-cooking grains (such as millet, teff, quinoa, amaranth and buckwheat) in a pre-heated thermos bottle and pour in boiling water to cover. Let stand overnight, and you and your breakfast will be ready to go in the morning.

Our quality of life depends on the quality of our food. We can only expect superior health when our food is healthful, and bursting with vital energy and abundant nutrients. Starting your day with a wholesome, nourishing breakfast goes a long way in caring for your health and that of your family.

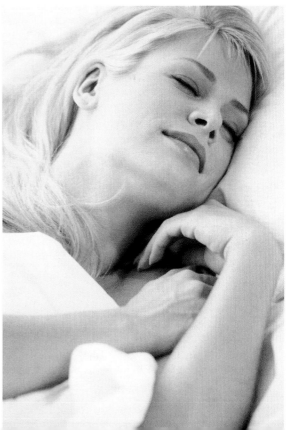

Start your day with a wholesome, nourishing breakfast by setting it up to prepare while you sleep.

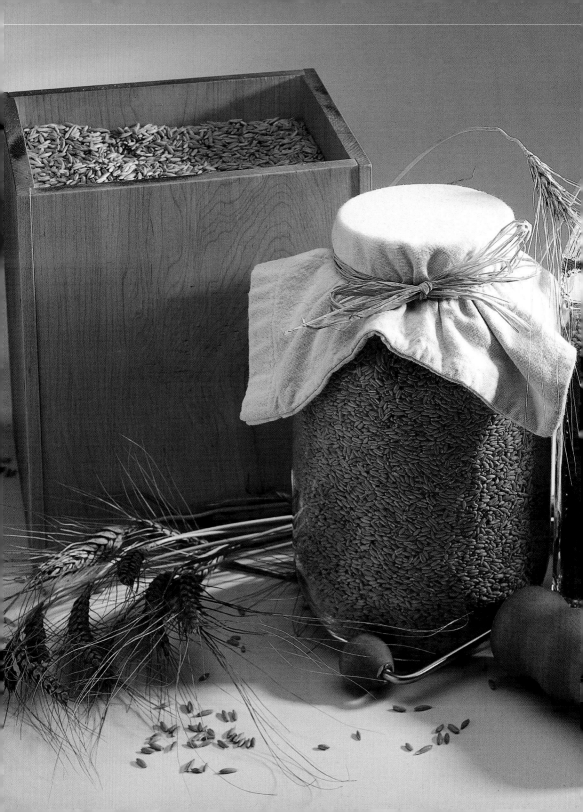

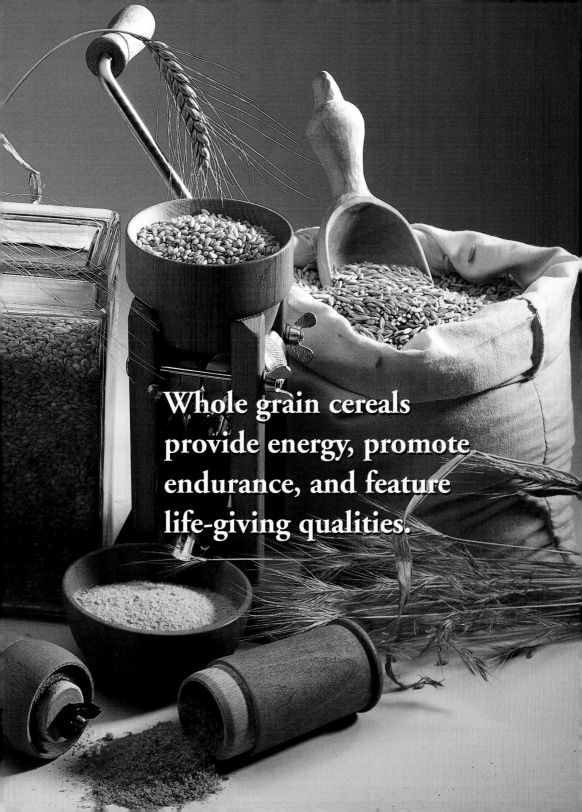

Whole grain cereals
provide energy, promote
endurance, and feature
life-giving qualities.

Banana Oats

Among the cereal grains, oats can be regularly eaten raw due to their healthy high fat and unique fiber content. The Goralen people in the Carpathian Mountains of Poland have enjoyed raw oatmeal for generations.

½ **cup** (125 ml) **whole oat groats**

½ **cup** (125 ml) **water**

¼ **cup** (60 ml) **unpasteurized yogurt**

1-2 tsp unpasteurized honey (optional)

2 tbsp flax seed oil

1 tbsp lemon juice, freshly squeezed

2 bananas, sliced or mashed

1 tbsp fresh pumpkin seeds

Grind the whole oat groats to a fine or medium meal. In a bowl, soak the oatmeal in the water at room temperature for 15 to 30 minutes.

Stir in yogurt, honey, and flax seed oil. Squeeze lemon juice over top of banana and combine with the oatmeal mixture. Sprinkle with pumpkin seeds and serve.

Serves 2

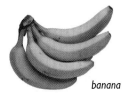

banana

The oat flakes found in stores are usually steam-rolled, a heat-treatment that supposedly extends their shelf life by about four months. Taste a few oat flakes by chewing them thoroughly: if a sweet, pleasant taste fills your mouth, they are okay to buy. Any bitterness indicates rancidity and will give your liver a tough time.

You can very easily roll your own flakes from whole oat groats. Even if you don't own a grain mill or flaker, any blender will turn out oatmeal because oat groats are very soft compared to wheat berries. The finer the oatmeal the easier it is for small children and elderly people to digest it.

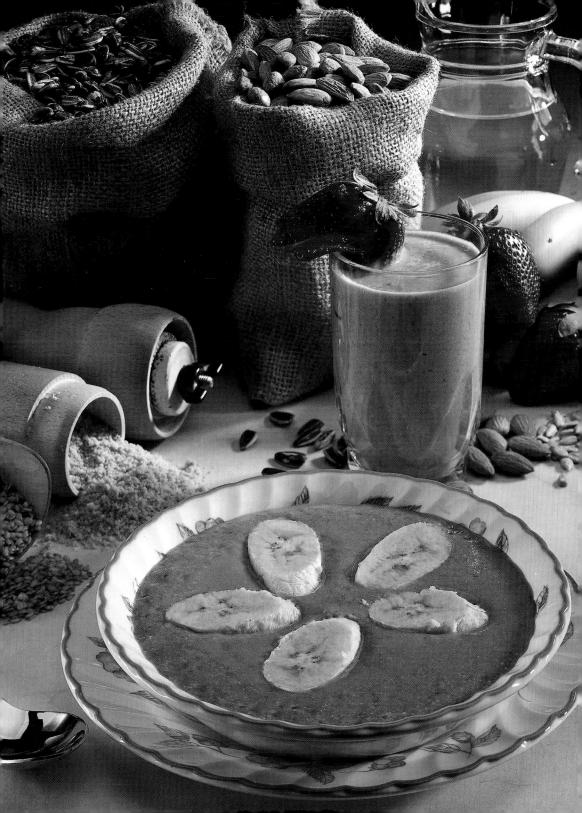

Seed Shake

This instant breakfast will really shake you up in the morning. Just add water and these little seeds get pretty busy during the night while you sleep. Water triggers a myriad of reactions, producing, for example, substantial amounts of vitamins C and E. The reward is an abundance of nutrients including essential fatty acids and lots of calcium, all offered in an easily digestible form. This shake only takes a few minutes to assemble, and after drinking it, you'll be wide awake and well prepared to enjoy a new day.

2 tbsp raw almonds

2 tbsp sunflower seeds, hulled

2 tbsp sesame seeds, unhulled

2 tbsp flax seeds

1-2 cups (250-500 ml) **water, at room temperature, divided**

1 cup (125 ml) **fresh or frozen berries**

1-2 tsp unpasteurized honey

Soak almonds and sunflower seeds in 1 cup (250 ml) of water. In another bowl, soak sesame seeds in ½ cup (125 ml) of water. In a separate bowl, soak the flax seeds in ¼ cup (60 ml) of water. Let the seeds sit at room temperature overnight or for 6 to 10 hours.

Drain the almonds, sunflower and sesame seeds (remove the hulls) and rinse them thoroughly. Place the rinsed seeds, flax seeds with soak water, berries and honey in a blender; liquefy. Add more water until you reach a desired consistency. Serve immediately in tall glasses.

Serves 2

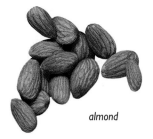

almond

Drinking the almond and seed soak waters is not recommended because they contain a lot of undesirable bitter substances. In contrast, the soak water of flax seeds turns into a jelly-like pudding that contains all the mucilage you want to guarantee regular bowel movements. If you find separate bowls for soaking too complicated, simply substitute the soaked flax seeds with 2 tablespoons of freshly ground flaxmeal.

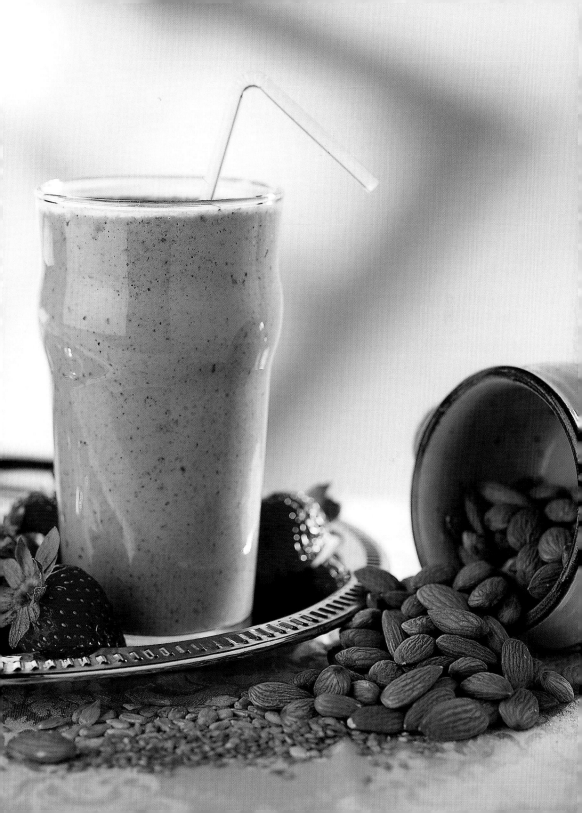

Bircher Muesli

Swiss medical doctor Maximilian Bircher-Benner practiced holistic medicine at the turn of the century. Instead of calorie counting and nutritional analysis, he simply recommended consuming as much sun-ripened raw food as possible. Inspired by a farmer's tradition in the Swiss Alps, he came up with a fresh apple breakfast to cure his dyspeptic and constipated contemporaries. The following recipe is based on his original formula–fruity, fresh and fabulous.

2 tbsp whole oat groats

¼ cup (60 ml) **water**

2 tbsp raw almonds

2 tbsp lemon juice, freshly squeezed

2 tbsp unpasteurized yogurt

1 tsp unpasteurized honey, optional

2-3 ripe apples

Flake the oat groats, place them in a bowl and soak them in the water for 15 to 30 minutes at room temperature. Grind or chop the almonds; set aside.

In a separate bowl, combine lemon juice, yogurt and honey. Grate the apples into the lemon sauce. Stir in rolled oats and sprinkle with ground almonds. Serve immediately.

Serves 2

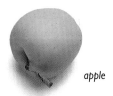

apple

Muesli Dessert
Muesli isn't just a breakfast food. Special occasions call for an elegant dessert consisting of muesli layered with blueberries, sour cherries or pineapple chunks and topped with whipping cream (or nut cream topping) and fresh walnuts.

Friendly Bacteria
A whole host of friendly bacteria works in your intestines to help you stay on top of things. Fermented food contains friendly bacteria and additional vitamins to support you and your intestinal flora. Always choose fermented milk products like unpasteurized yogurt and kefir over plain cow's milk, which is relatively difficult to digest. If you have access to fresh and healthy milk, make your own yogurt. Otherwise make sure the yogurt you buy is made from only bacterial cultures and milk, not so-called milk ingredients. Raw sauerkraut and freshly brewed rejuvelac are other popular fermented choices.

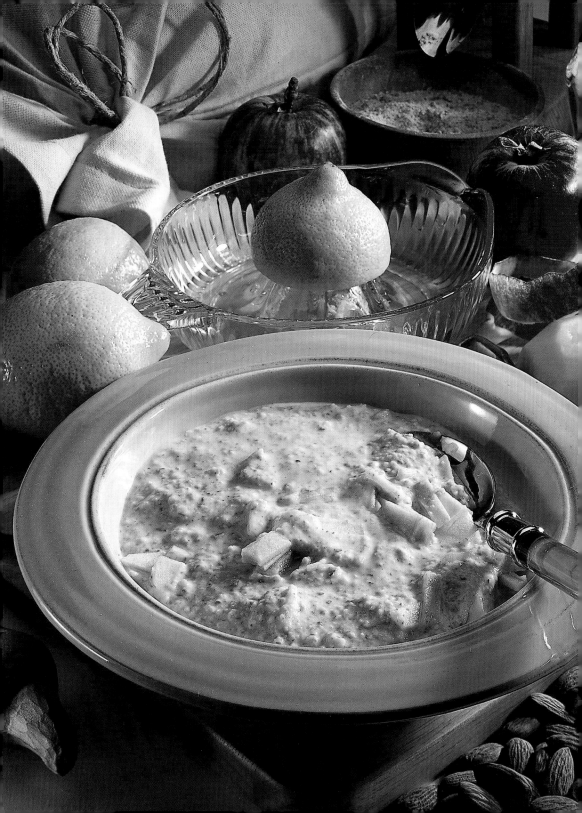

Carrot Muesli

Muesli can be fresh and satisfying. Simply roll your oats along with the flax seeds first thing in the morning. And while they soak a little bit (for easier digestion) you can get dressed. Or, if you want to take your time and you love to chew, don't bother soaking the oat flakes. However, those with a sensitive digestive system, such as little children, elderly people, and all the stressed souls in-between, will benefit from soaking. In particular, it is preferable to soak flakes of hardier grains, such as wheat, rye, and barley for 1 to 6 hours.

½ **cup** (125 ml) **oat flakes**

¼ **cup** (60 ml) **cold water**

½ **cup** (125 ml) **yogurt or almond milk**

1 tbsp flax seeds, freshly ground

1 tsp unpasteurized honey

1/2 tsp anise, ground

1 medium carrot

2 ripe apples

2-3 tbsp hazelnuts, freshly chopped

In a bowl, soak oat flakes in cold water for 15 to 30 minutes.

In a separate bowl, combine yogurt, flax, honey and anise. Grate carrots (finely) and apples (coarsely) into the mixture then add oat flakes and mix thoroughly. Sprinkle with hazelnuts and serve.

Serves 2

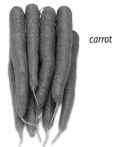

carrot

Flax Seeds
This little seed has lots to offer. It supplies soothing and cleansing mucilage and more importantly bursts with omega-3 essential fatty acid, making flax extremely valuable for human nutrition. Make sure you have enough liquid with flax because it absorbs a lot of water. Improperly chewed, whole flax seeds tend to escape digestion, so they're better freshly ground in a poppy seed mill or coffee grinder. Store this meal in an airtight glass jar and it will keep for a week in your refrigerator.

Flax Oil
Fresh flax oil is hard to come by because its delicate ingredients deteriorate so quickly. You can order several bottles at a time directly from the oil mill or health food store and then put them in the freezer where they'll keep for up to 6 months. Take out a fresh bottle each week and enjoy. For more information on the powerful health benefits of flax, see *Fantastic Flax* written by publisher Siegfried Gursche (*alive* Natural Health Guide #1, 1999).

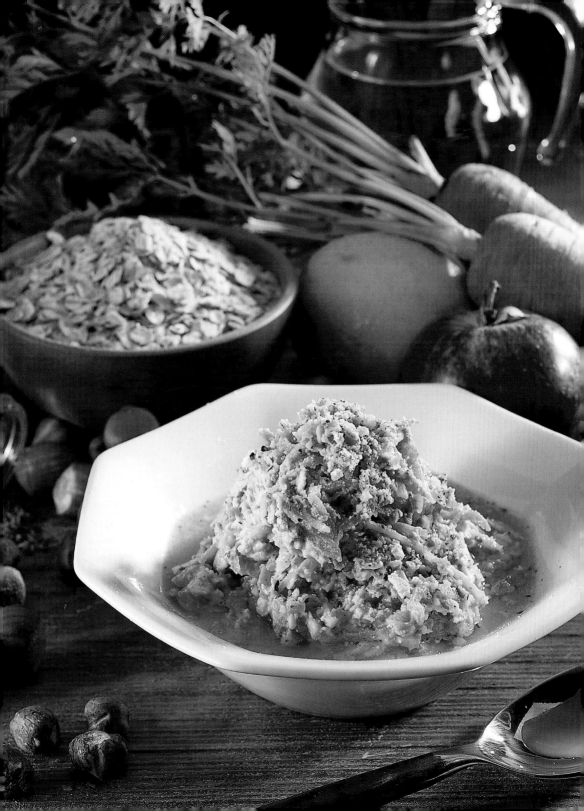

Muesli with Whipping Cream

Muesli does not need to be mushy. You can elegantly layer the grain flakes with blueberries, sour cherries, or pineapple chunks and top it all with whipping cream of your choice for special occasions.

1 cup (100 g) **oat flakes**

½ cup (125 ml) **water**

2 cups (250 g) **fresh or frozen blueberries**

2 tbsp natural sugar

1-2 tbsp lemon juice, freshly squeezed

¼ tsp vanilla, ground

½ tsp cinnamon, ground

½ tsp freshly grated ginger root

¼ cup (60 ml) **whipping cream**

¼ cup (60 ml) **unpasteurized yogurt**

2-3 tbsp raw walnuts

Soak oat flakes in cold water for about 15-30 minutes.

Meanwhile, season the blueberries with natural sugar, lemon juice, vanilla, cinnamon and frshly grated ginger. Cover and let stand.

Whisk cool whipping cream until it holds its shape. Now fold in yogurt and some ground anise. Any nut cream topping will taste as delicious as old-fashioned whipping cream.

Serve this muesli on plates: first a layer of soaked oat flakes, next a layer of the seasoned blueberries, and all of this topped with wipping cream and sprinkled around with chopped walnuts, Serve immediately.

Serves 2-3

Natural Sugar
Natural sugar crystals may be equally substituted for the white sugar called in your recipes. There are many types of natural sugar crystals on the market. Some are superior to others simply because of the way they're made. I use either Sucanat or Rapadura, which is dried cane juice and totally unrefined. Unlike the process used to make white refined sugar, the process used to make these natural sugars preserves the natural rich flavor and nutrition, without preservatives or additives, and actually results in a lower level of sucrose than refined sugar.

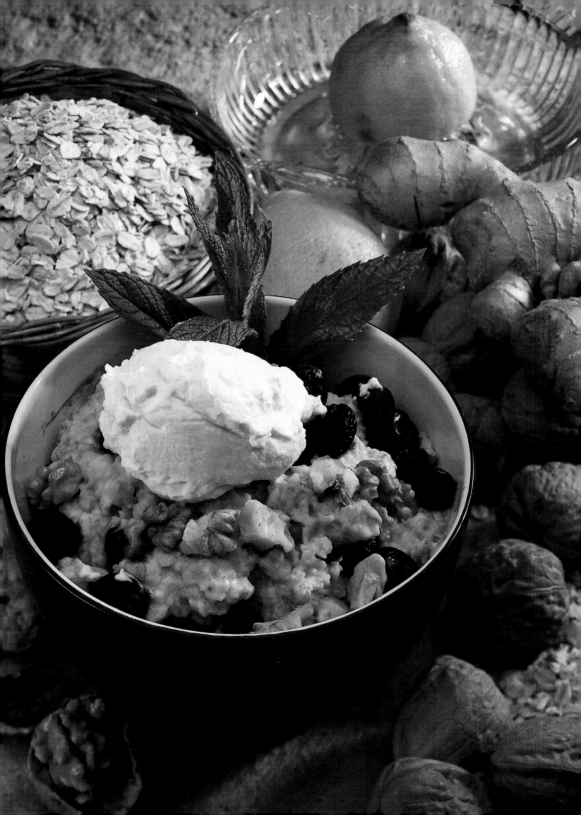

Sun Sprout Cereal

Ancient cultures considered wheat a divine gift. In Persia, wheat was synonymous with the sun. The founder of the old Iranian religion, Zoroaster, taught his followers to eat the fruit of the field, that is wheat, for its life- and light-giving qualities. Sprouted wheat cleanses and lights up one's life because a whole bunch of protein, enzymes and vitamins are newly synthesized during the sprouting process. However, digesting it requires a lot of internal heat and so sensitive or stressed people can experience shivers of cold when eating it. In this case, simply start with small amounts or try just its juice–raw grain milk.

2-3 tbsp soft wheat kernels

1-1 ½ cups (250-375 ml) **water, for soaking, divided**

1-2 tbsp sunflower seeds, hulled

6 dried apricots

In a bowl, soak soft wheat kernels in 1 cup (250 ml) of water for about 10 hours.

Pour off soak water and let sprout for 2 to 3 days, rinsing with fresh water twice daily until the shoots are about as long as the kernels. (If only half the wheat kernels sprout, discard them and find better quality wheat.)

In the meantime, soak the sunflower seeds in ¼ cup (60 ml) water overnight. In a separate bowl, soak the dried apricots in ¼ cup (60 ml) water overnight.

Thoroughly rinse and drain wheat sprouts. In a blender, purée apricots in their soak water. Add wheat sprouts and blend with apricots, or combine them whole. Thoroughly rinse sunflower seeds and sprinkle them on top of the apricot-wheat sprout mixture.

Serves 1

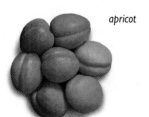

apricot

Many types of wheat are available. For a sprouted breakfast cereal soft wheat, kamut, and spelt are most desirable because unlike hard wheat, their bran layers are less tough and they taste sweeter. Rye sprouts are another good choice. Simply purée with yogurt or soaked nuts and enjoy a heavenly, creamy experience.

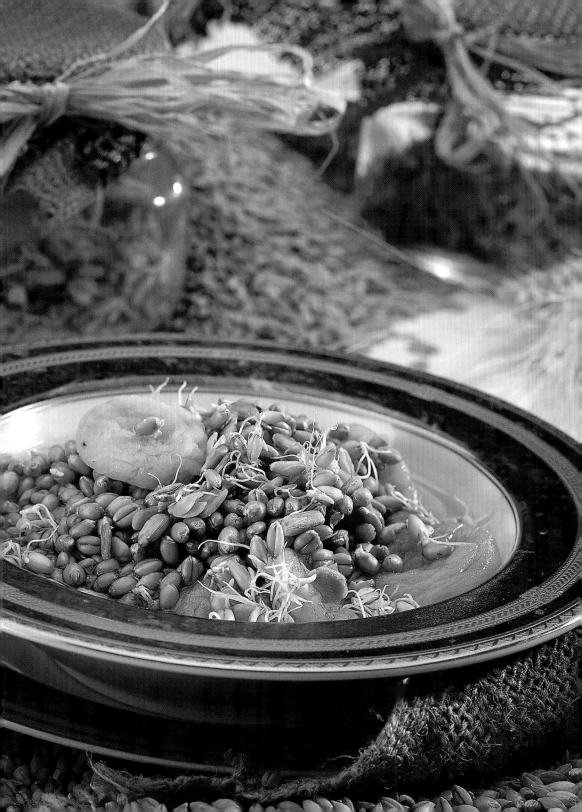

Kollath Breakfast

Dr. Werner Kollath was one of the pioneers of the health food movement in Germany, coining the phrase "Let our food be as natural as possible." He also came up with a fresh breakfast idea. The grain of your choice only needs to be freshly ground, and if you choose oats, this raw cereal can be eaten year round. As far as other grains are concerned, amazing cleansing reactions can be triggered, but they should be taken with caution in this raw formula because they can easily overtax a fragile person, particularly a child.

¼ **cup** (60 ml) **whole cereal grains such as oats, soft wheat, or rye**

¼ **cup** (60 ml) **cool water**

2 tbsp unpasteurized yogurt or almond butter

1 tsp unpasteurized honey

1-2 tsp lemon juice, freshly squeezed

1 ripe apple

1 tbsp raw hazelnuts, freshly chopped

Freshly grind the cereal grain of your choice or a combination of them to a coarse meal. Add the water, cover with a plate and let soak at cool room temperature for 1 to 10 hours, or overnight.

The next morning, combine lemon juice, yogurt (or almond butter) and honey in a bowl. Grate the apple into the lemon sauce. Stir in the wholemeal and sprinkle hazelnuts over top. Serve immediately (before the apple turns brown).

Serves 1

lemon

Ripe Fruit
Any claims about the healing powers of raw food assumes that the fruit in question is fully ripe, and ideally picked shortly before consumption. Eating unripe fruit leads to discomfort, diarrhea or stomach upset. It is the plant's way of discouraging us from devouring its seeds before it had a chance to develop them completely for successful reproduction.

It's worth searching for local fruit that's been grown organically and allowed to develop its full potential. Anything coming from further afield often isn't given the time to mature. For instance, you want to look for apples with intense colors of red, orange, and yellow on the outside (don't be fooled by glossy synthetic waxes) and dark-colored seeds inside. Bananas are usually picked unripe and they should be eaten only after they turn a bright yellow and no hint of green remains.

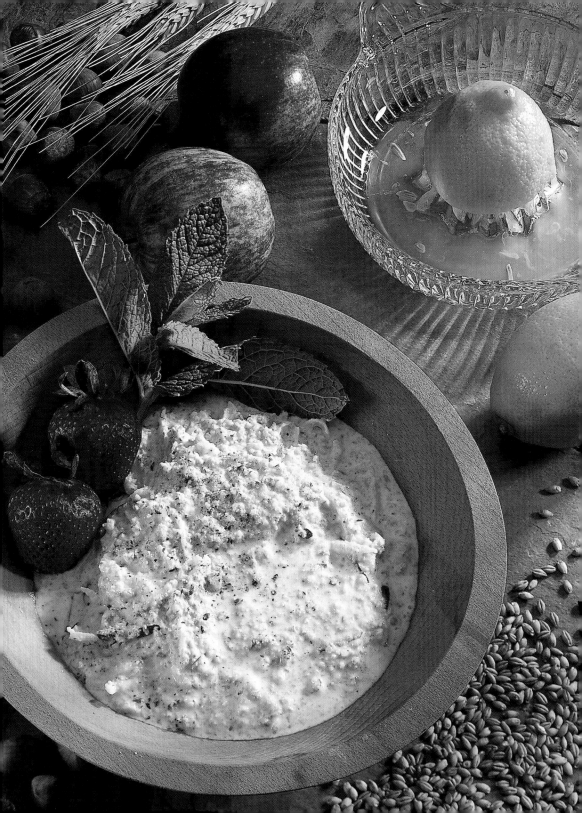

Cornmeal Mush

The native American version of the universal dish—mush—is based on corn. The first European settlers discovered its nourishing qualities quickly, especially during long, cold winters. Corn comes in a rainbow of colors such as white, yellow, and blue. Blue corn surprises with its striking color and also its abundance of nutrients, including an extra helping of minerals due to its heirloom descent. However, when the smell of your freshly ground corn reminds you of paint thinner, you better reach for popcorn, which is usually fresh and works just as well in this recipe.

1 cup (250 ml) **yellow, white, or blue corn**

1 cup (250 ml) **water, for soaking**

3-4 cups (750 ml-1 l) **water, for cooking**

Dash sea salt

Agave nector or raw honey, to taste (optional)

Grind the corn kernels into a coarse or fine meal. In a bowl, soak the cornmeal in the water for ½ to 1 hour—the coarser the cornmeal, the longer the soak period.

Bring fresh water and a generous dash of salt to a boil in a pot. Add the cornmeal and stir for 5 to 10 minutes or until it completely dissolves and starts to thicken. Turn down the heat, cover and let stand for 30 minutes.

Serve warm in breakfast bowls and drizzle with agave nectar or raw honey if you like.

Serves 4

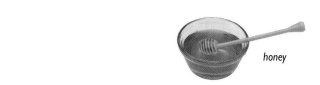

honey

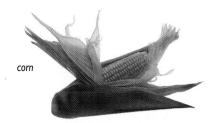

corn

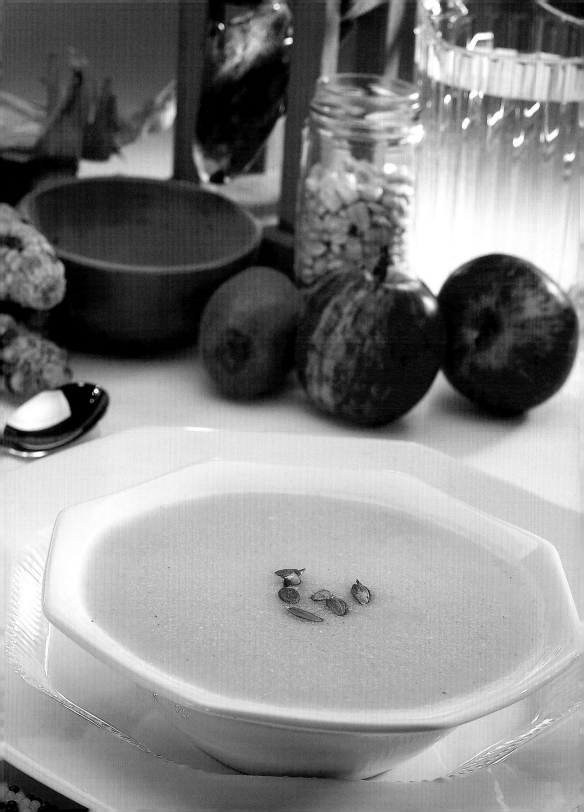

Spelt Gruel

One thousand years ago a visionary abbess from Southern Germany, Hildegard von Bingen, recommended spelt gruel as the ultimate breakfast dish. In a region where people are confronted with chilly mornings half the year, this proved to be worthwhile advice.

1 cup (250 ml) **whole spelt kernels**

1 cup (250 ml) **water, for soaking**

3 cups (750 ml) **water, for cooking**

Dash sea salt

½ tsp ground anise seed or fennel seed (optional)

Grind the spelt kernels into a coarse or fine meal. In a bowl, soak the speltmeal in the water for ½ to 1 hour (the coarser the speltmeal, the longer the soak period).

Bring fresh water and a generous dash of salt to a boil in a pot. Add anise for a sweet flavor if you choose. Add spelt and stir for 5 to 10 minutes or until it completely dissolves and starts to thicken. Turn down the heat, cover and let stand for 30 minutes.

Serve warm in breakfast bowls.

Serves 3 to 4

Spelt is a highly nutritious grain providing more crude fiber and more protein than wheat. It also contains all eight of the essential amino acids that the body requires for proper cell maintenance. Spelt is also easily digested–in fact, it is better tolerated by the body than any other grain.

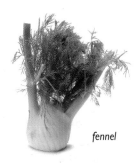

fennel

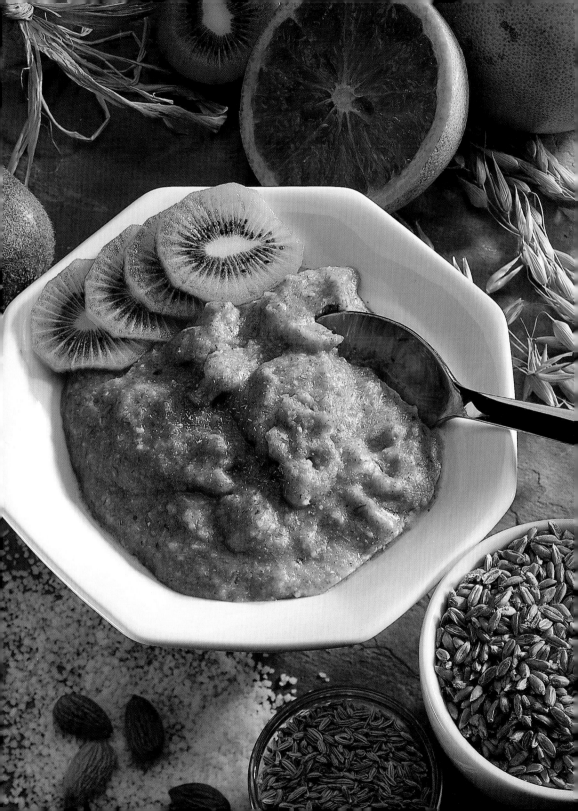

Rye Porridge

The Scots always know how to stir their pot so that their porridge turns out golden, smooth, and creamy with a lovely warm comforting aroma. I've varied the traditional oat porridge with rye, another hardy grain that spoils us with a surprising creaminess.

1 cup (250 ml) **rye kernels**

1 cup (250 ml) **cold water**

2-3 cups (500-750 ml) **water**

¼ tsp whole sea salt

4-6 tbsp fresh flax seed oil or cultured butter

1 cup (250 ml) **whole milk or nut milk**

Grind the rye kernels to a coarse to medium meal. In a bowl, soak the coarse ryemeal in the cold water. Cover and let stand for 30 to 60 minutes, or overnight.

Heat fresh water and the salt in a pot. Add soaked ryemeal and stir until porridge starts to thicken. Turn heat off and cover. Post-soak in a warm place for ½ to 1 hour.

Pour porridge into bowls, drizzle with flax seed oil (or dot with butter), pour milk over top and serve hot.

Serves 4

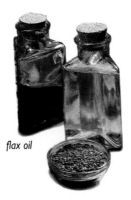

flax oil

If you're in a rush in the mornings, grind the rye the previous afternoon for pre-soaking, cook it in the evening, and let it post-soak all night in a warm place. If desired, gently reheat the porridge the next morning and add more hot water until the desired consistency. If you find the porridge too thick, the next time try adding an extra cup of water right at the beginning.

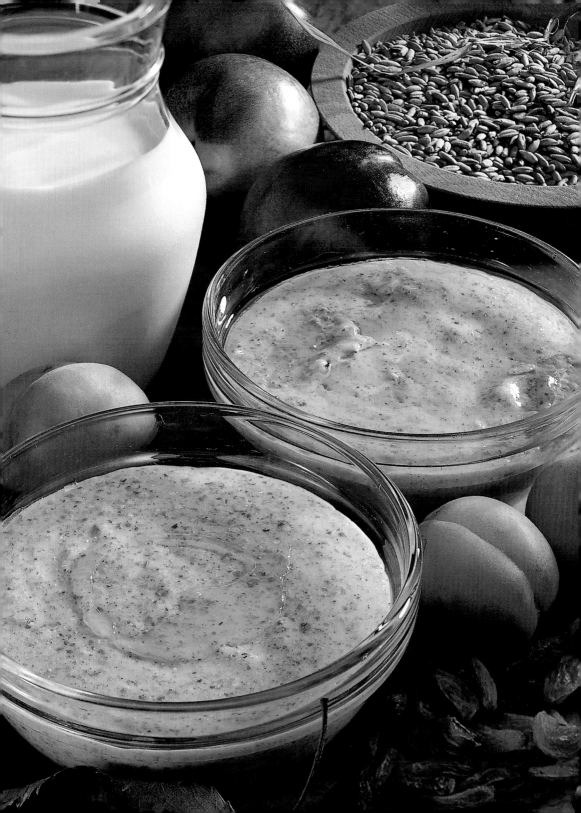

Cream of Rice

Ironically, cream of wheat is sold with the image of being the cream of the crop. Nothing could be further from the truth. You're actually offered only the leftover after the inner part of the wheat kernel has been "purified." For a truly creamy experience, it's not necessary to sacrifice taste by throwing out all the bran layers, not to mention all the nutrients. Start with a fully flavored whole grain such as kamut, rice, corn, or millet and finely grind it into flour.

⅓ **cup** (80 ml) **long grain or basmati brown rice**

½ **cup** (125 ml) **cold water, for soaking**

1 **cup** (250 ml) **water, for cooking**

¼ **tsp cinnamon**

Dash whole sea salt

½ **cup** (125 ml) **milk**

2 **tbsp freshly squeezed lemon juice, optional**

2 **tbsp fresh flax seed oil**

2 **tsp unpasteurized honey**

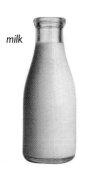

milk

Grind brown rice into a fine to medium flour and stir into the cold water; let soak for 15 minutes.

Heat fresh water with the cinnamon and salt in a double boiler or pot. Add soaked rice flour and stir until mixture is creamy and starts to thicken. Turn heat down to low, cover and let stand for 10 to 15 minutes.

Stir in warm milk (don't heat milk above 140ºF/60ºC) then turn off the heat, place an unbleached cotton/paper towel under the lid and let the mixture post-soak for ½ hour longer.

Pour mixture into a large bowl and whisk until desired creaminess. Stir in flax seed oil and rejuvelac (or lemon juice). Add honey when the cream of rice is warm, otherwise it will turn very liquidy and the precious enzymes in the honey will be lost. Serve with freshly sliced fruit if you like.

Serves 2

Variations: To add a nuttier flavor and eliminate pre-soak time, substitute the unsoaked rice with dry-toasted brown rice, spelt, kamut, oats or whatever grain you like. Once you have dry-toasted the grain of your choice, you can always grind a batch ahead of time and it will keep for up to 4 months. For a variation of the above recipe, simply measure ½ cup (125 ml) of dry-toasted flour, mix it with cold water and pour it in boiling water. Even though pre-soaking isn't required, you must mix the flour with water before you add it to the boiling water, otherwise you end up with a lumpy mess.

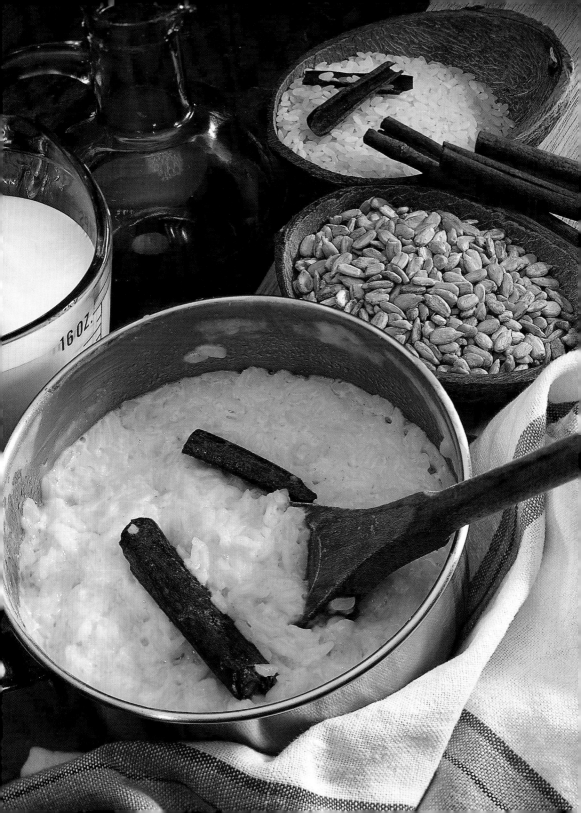

Golden Congee

Congee is a specialty that is eaten from Japan to Persia. The English word "congee" is borrowed from the Tamil language meaning "rice water." You simply take a little rice, millet, oats, amaranth or whatever whole grain you like and boil it in lots of water (six to eight times the amount of grain). The Chinese say the longer it simmers the more powerful it will be to harmonize your digestion.

½ cup (125 ml) **millet, hulled**

3 cups (750 ml) **water**

Dash sea salt

Rinse the millet in several changes of water until the water runs clear. If desired, soak millet in ½ cup (125 ml) of cold water for about 15 minutes for better digestibility. Bring water, salt and millet to a boil in a pot, double boiler, or rice cooker (in the evening, for instance). Turn down the heat to low and simmer for 1 hour or until most of the water is absorbed. You can also keep this soup warm overnight and served it first thing the next morning.

Serve hot in breakfast bowls along with raw sauerkraut or any other vegetable of your choice.

Variation: If you prefer traditional rice, take 3 ½ cups (875 ml) water per ½ cup (60 ml) short grain brown rice and simmer it for 1 ½ to 2 hours.

Serves 2 to 3

Hulled millet tends to be rancid by the time it reaches your local health food store. If you're unable to locate freshly hulled millet, pour hot water over the millet to wash off the rancid germ oils. Drain and rinse several times with cold water until the water runs clear. Freshly hulled millet only needs rinsing under cold water.

Chinese prefer eating congee with vegetables, no matter what time of day. Try it with bok choy, lightly sautéed with minced ginger, sesame seed oil (or olive oil) and soy sauce. The Japanese enjoy their congee with pickled carrot or daikon.

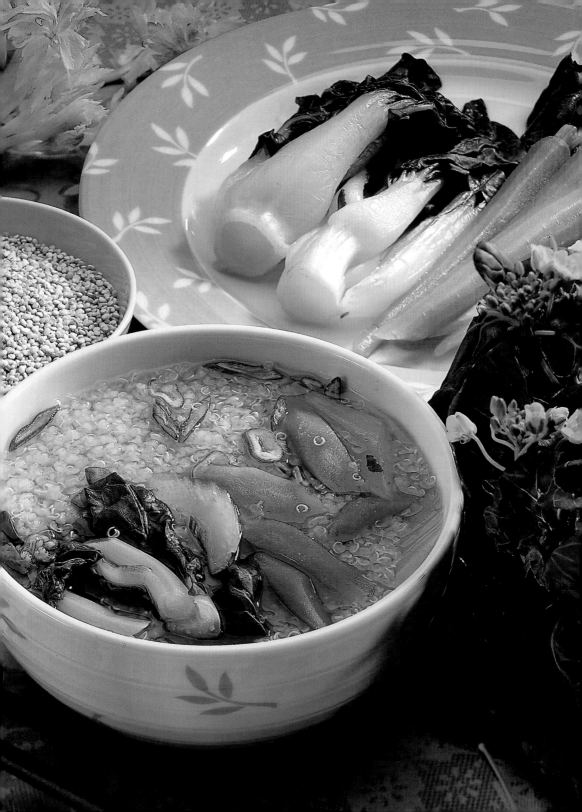

Tzampa

In the high altitudes of Tibet where life is harsh yet beautiful, nomads trade their gathered salt mainly for barley. This barley is dry-toasted then ground into a flour, the so-called tzampa.

1 cup (125 ml) **hull-less barley or spelt**

2 cups (500 ml) **water**

Toast larger amounts in the oven 170° to 210°F (80° to 100°C) for about 1 hour. This process is gentler and requires you to stir only once or twice.

In a bowl, soak barley kernels in the water for about 15 minutes. Rinse and drain then cover the moist barley with a plate. Let stand at room temperature for 3 to 10 hours.

Once the barley feels almost dry to the touch, dry-toast it over medium heat in a cast-iron or heavy-bottom skillet for 15 minutes or until it turns a golden hue and fills your kitchen with a fragrant aroma. Stir constantly to prevent burning, and avoid roasting.

Let the dry-toasted barley cool then grind it into a flour. This tzampa will keep in a covered wooden box or airtight glass jar for several weeks without much loss in nutrients. Freshly ground tzampa tastes almost like walnuts.

Tzampa Tea

Tibetan nomads traditionally have green or black tea in the morning mixed with fresh yak's milk, aged butter and a dash of salt. After drinking half a cup of tea, tzampa is poured into remaining tea and the mixture formed into little bite-size pieces of dough then eaten.

1 cup (250 ml) **hot tea of your choice** (such as green, linden blossom or rose petal tea)

½-1 tsp cultured butter or flax seed oil

Dash whole sea salt

½ cup (125 ml) **tzampa**

In a bowl or large cup, combine tea, butter, and salt. Stir in tzampa until the consistency is to your liking. The given recipe makes a porridge-like gruel that you can eat with a spoon. However, you can always add more tzampa and enjoy it by each delicious morsel.

Serves 1

Tzampa Cream

Instantly whip up a bowl of cream with tzampa. You can stir tzampa into any liquid, it doesn't need to be hot. Nut milk, for example, also tastes great in the following recipe.

1 cup (250 ml) **unpasteurized whole milk yogurt**

½ cup (125 ml) **tzampa**

Dash sea salt, optional

2 medium-size ripe apples, cored and diced

1 tbsp lemon juice, freshly squeezed

1 tbsp unpasteurized honey

20 raw almonds, soaked 6 to 10 hours

In a bowl, combine yogurt and tzampa. Add a dash of salt to bring out the nutty flavor even more. If preferred, let the tzampa soak for a little while.

In a separate bowl, combine apples, lemon juice, and honey. Pour tzampa cream over the apples, sprinkle almonds over top and serve.

Serves 2

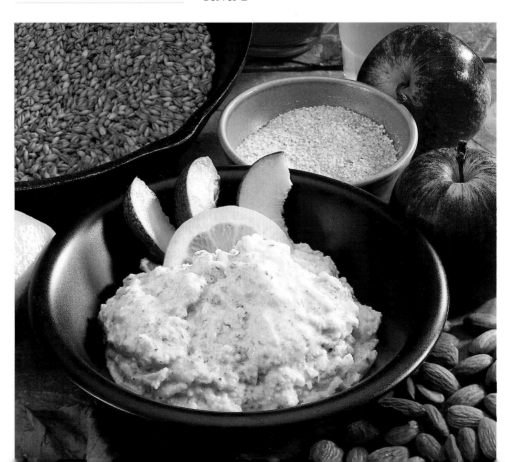

Fancy Granola

As soon as you add fat to your granola, you're moving away from everyday breakfast cereals and creating a snack or dessert. By taking extra care, however, you can still turn out a wholesome food. First, choose a fat that can handle a bit of heat such as unrefined coconut oil or ghee (clarified butter). Never use butter because the milk solids in it will simply burn. Incorporate some water to bake more than roast, then toast at a low temperature, that is below 300ºF (150ºC), in order to keep the vitamin B complex in your cereal flakes intact. Other than that, combine your favorite flakes and nuts to your liking.

5 cups (1.25 l) **oat flakes**

1 cup (250 ml) **walnuts, hulled and chopped**

½ cup (125 ml) **sunflower seeds, unhulled** (optional)

½ cup (125 ml) **pumpkin seeds** (optional)

¼ cup (60 ml) **water**

1 cup (250 ml) **maple syrup or barley malt**

½ cup (125 ml) **unrefined coconut oil or ghee**

Dash whole sea salt

1 tsp cinnamon, ground

1 tsp anise, ground

Oven Temperature:	250ºF (120ºC)
Rack Placement:	center
Dry-Toasting Time:	1 hour

Preheat the oven to 250°F (120°C). Line 2 large baking sheets with unbleached baking paper; set aside.

In a large bowl, combine oats, walnuts, and the seeds of your choice.

In a saucepan, gently warm the water, maple syrup, coconut oil, and salt over medium heat until the maple syrup dissolves completely. Pour liquid over granola and combine ingredients thoroughly.

Spread mixture onto the baking sheets and place on the center rack in the oven for about 1 hour, stirring once after ½ hour to ensure even toasting.

Pour granola into a bowl. Add spices when still warm. Let cool completely then place in airtight glass jars and store in a cool place. It will keep for about 4 months.

This granola is great on top of yogurt, kefir, buttermilk, nut milk and the like. Any desired dried fruit should be added after toasting.

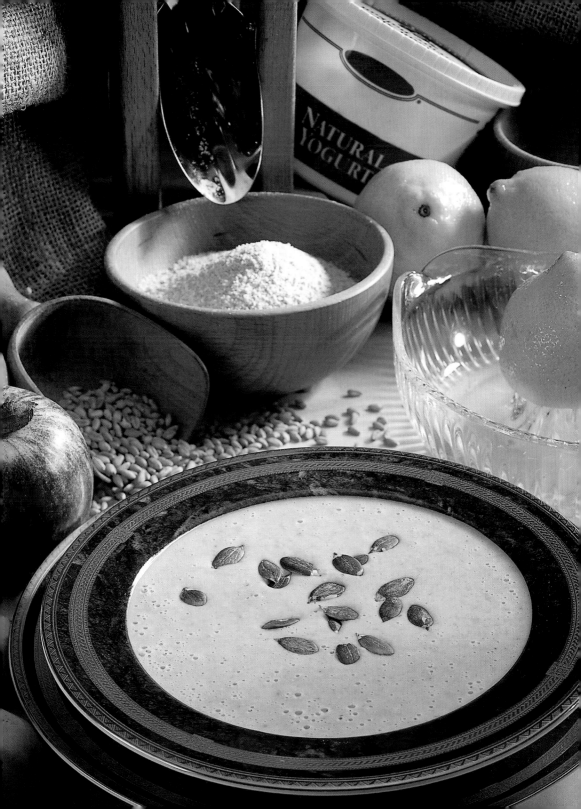

Buckwheat Crispies

Usually, buckwheat is either loved or loathed. People in Northern and Eastern Europe didn't have much of a choice in the past, enjoying their buckwheat as either gruel or pancake. Buckwheat also lends itself to this heavenly crunchy experience.

1 cup (250 ml) **buckwheat groats, hulled**

Bake larger amounts in the oven. Spread 2 cups (500 ml) soaked and strained buckwheat groats on a large baking sheet lined with unbleached baking paper and dry-toast at 170° to 210°F (80° to 100°C) for about 1 hour.

Dry toasting: Rinse buckwheat groats until water runs clear. Drain and place in a strainer for 1 hour or until they are almost dry to the touch. You do not want to skip this first step because it makes for a naturally sweeter taste.

Heat a heavy-bottom skillet and dry-toast buckwheat groats, stirring occasionally to prevent burning, for 10 to 20 minutes or until buckwheat turns golden red and a fragrant aroma fills your kitchen. Remove from heat and spread on a plate to cool. Avoid roasting the buckwheat.

Variation: Substitute the buckwheat with millet.

Buckwheat Pancakes

1 ½ cups (375 ml) **buckwheat, dry-toasted**

¼ cup (60 ml) **hot water**

¼ cup (60 ml) **cream**

1 free-range egg

1 ½ tsp unpasteurized honey

pinch sea salt

2 drops olive oil

3 tbsp olive oil (for frying)

Follow above directions for dry-toasting buckwheat. Grind it into a semi-fine flour. Add the hot water and soak for one and-a-half hours. Once soaked, add the cream, egg, honey, sea salt, and olive oil, and mix thoroughly. Heat the olive oil in a pan or on a griddle and drop approximately ⅛ cup of batter onto pan and fry both sides until brown. These dense, filling, and nutritious pancakes are both tasty and satisfying.

Serves 2

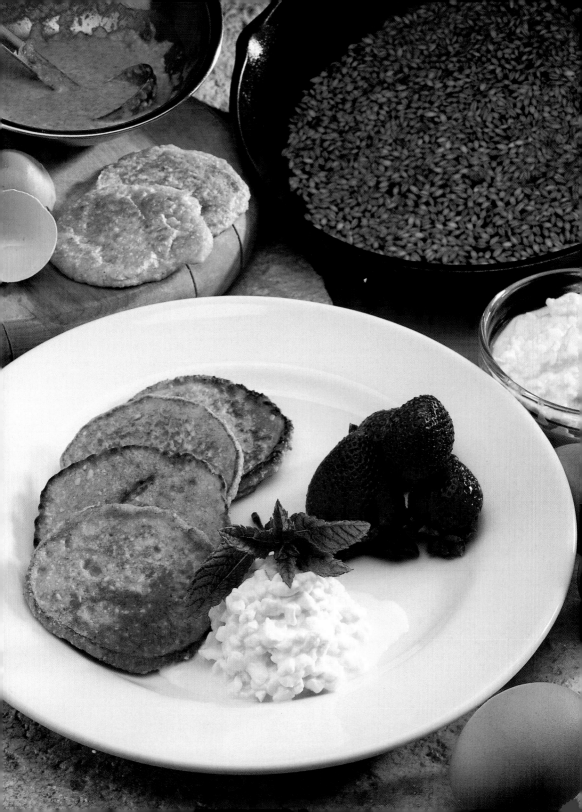

Grain Suppliers

Please note, no matter where you get your grains from, you must always check for insect and mold infestation as well as rancidity. I encourage you to ask for harvest and processing dates. It is also worth inquiring about germination rates even though your supplier often won't be able to tell you.

Local Health Food Stores

You can usually find quite a selection of whole grains at your local health food store and receive a 10 to 15 percent discount when ordering a 55- or 25-pound bag.

Organic Resource Guide

The most comprehensive directory of organic agriculture listing farmers, mills, wholesalers and other related resources from all over Canada. Available from the publisher for $16.95 (by cheque).
Canadian Organic Growers
Box 6408, Station "J"
Ottawa, ON K2A 3Y6

Grain Mills and Flakers:

bio supply ltd.

6-310 Goldstream Avenue
Victoria, BC V9B 2W3
Tel: (250) 478-3244
Fax: (250) 478-3057
Supplies: Schnitzer's Grain Mills from Germany-hand and electric mills

Berry Hill Limited

75 Burwell Road
St. Thomas, ON N5P 3R5
Tel: (519) 631-0480
toll-free: 1-800-668-3072
Fax: (519) 631-8935
Free catalogue available
Selection of various hand and electric mills: Corona, Country Living Grain Mill, Retsel

Moulins - Abenakis - Milling

114 Rg St-Jean Nord
Ste-Claire, QC GOR 2V0
Tel: (418) 883-3688
Fax: (418) 883-2662
Free catalogue available
Supplies Hawo's Flour Mills from Germany-electric mills

Pfenning's Organic

RR #2
Baden, ON N0B 1G0
Tel: (519) 662-3468
Fax: (519) 662-4083
Email: pfennings.organic@sympatico.ca
Free catalogue available
Supplies SAMAP Grain Mills from France-hand and electric mills, and oat roller

Sovereignty Enterprises Ltd.

5755 Young Street
Halifax, NS B3K 1Z9
Tel: (902) 454-5454
Fax: (902) 454-5161
Supplies Hawo's Flour Mills from Germany-electric mills and oat roller

Gold Mine Natural Food Co.

3419 Hancock Street
San Diego, CA 92110-4307
Tel: (619) 296-8536
toll-free: 1-800-475-3663
Fax: (619) 296-9756
Email: goldmine@ix.netcom.com
Free catalogue available
Supplies Lehman's Hand Mill and Hawo's Electric Flour Mill

sources

Retsel Corporation
1567 East Highway 30
P.O. Box 37
McCammon, ID 83250
Tel: (208) 254-3737
toll-free: 1-800-854-8862
Fax: (208) 254-3325
Email: resales@retsel.com
Free catalogue available
Supplies Retsel Flour Mills from the
United States-hand and electric mills

Miracle Exclusives, Inc.
64 Seaview Blvd
Port Washington, NY 11050
Tel: (516) 621-3333
toll-free: 1-800-645-6360
Fax: (516) 621-1997
Email: miracle-exc@juno.com
Free catalogue available
Largest selection of hand mills,
electric mills and oat rollers:
Corona, Hawo's, Miracle Mill,
SAMAP, Schnitzer's and more

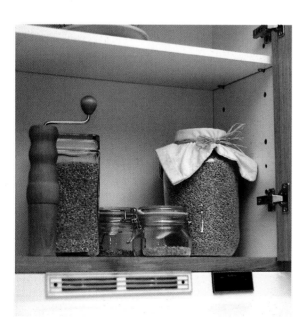

First published in 2000 by
alive **books**
7436 Fraser Park Drive
Burnaby BC V5J 5B9
(604) 435–1919
1–800–661–0303

© 2000 by *alive* books

Book Design:
   Liza Novecoski
Artwork:
   Terence Yeung
   Raymond Cheung
Food Styling:
   Fred Edrissi
Photography:
   Edmond Fong (recipe photos)
   Siegfried Gursche
Photo Editing:
   Sabine Edrissi-Bredenbrock
Editing:
   Sandra Tonn
   Julie Cheng

Canadian Cataloguing in
Publication Data

Gustavs, Katharina
   Super Breakfast Cereals

(*alive* natural health guides, 21
ISSN 1490-6503)
ISBN 1-55312-022-1

Printed in Canada

Revolutionary Health Books
alive Natural Health Guides

Each 64-page book focuses on a single subject, is written in easy-to-understand language and is lavishly illustrated with full color photographs.

New titles will be published every month in each of the four series.

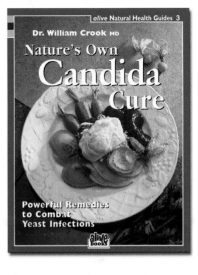

Series 1

Self Help Guides

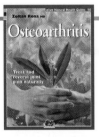
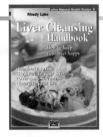

Series 2

Healthy Recipes

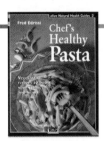
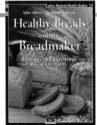
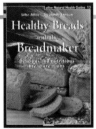

Series 3

Healing Foods & Herbs

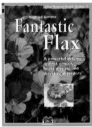
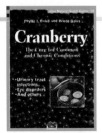

Series 4

Lifestyle & Alternative Treatments

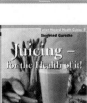
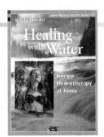

*Great gifts at
an amazingly
affordable price*

Cdn $9.95

US $8.95

UK £8.95

alive Natural Health Guides
are available in health and
nutrition centers and
in bookstores. For information
or to place orders please dial

1-800-663-6513

alive books

Vancouver
Canada